Keto Chaffle

Cookbook

50+ Easy, Appetizing and

Low Carbs Recipes to Live

Healthier

By Alice Allen

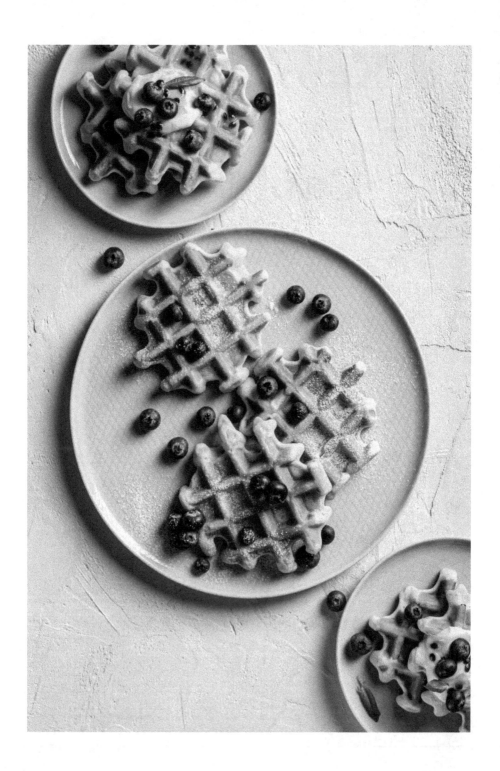

Table of Contents

Introduction

Chaffle

We present to you the "Chaffle" or "cheddar waffle", an extremely delicious waffle you can easily prepare at home, but made with egg and butter as base ingredients instead of grain, they are perfect to stay in ketosis as shredded cheese have no flour.

The high flour content in regular waffles adds a lot of carbohydrates that makes your body stop using fat as an energy resource, and consequently start accumulating it, due to spikes in your insulin levels caused by the carb intake.

This healthy food, that follow the ketogenic diet recommendations, will also keep you feeling full for a long time as they are high-fat and high-protein, preventing overeating, they are a great alternative for bread, perfect in their simplicity.

You can enjoy this mouth-watering dish in every meal of your day, there are countless combinations of low-carb ketogenic ingredients aviable, so it's easy to find a chaffle one to love!

Depending on how you serve them, they can be delicious sweet desserts, nutrient breakfast food or a quick snack, try them in sandiwhich, pizza and French toast variations!

The best option to make them is the Chaffle Maker, but you can prepare yourself one with a regular Waffle maker or even a nonstick saucepan.

Some people does not like the taste that comes from the egg as a base ingredients, here some tips on how to avoid too much eggy taste:
-Increase the sugar quantity
-Add milk powder
-Add Lime, lemon, or orange juice. Use a teaspoon of juice per 3 eggs
-Add some rind. Use quarter teaspoon per 3 eggs.
-Let chaffle cool completely
-Use egg whites instead of whole eggs

Note

➢ You can freeze them up for 3 to 5 days and then reheat them in a toaster oven, skillet, or conventional oven.

➢ You can also microwave for 30 to 60 seconds, but allow them to thaw before reheating.

- ➤ You can make two chaffles from a large egg and half a cup of shredded cheese.

- ➤ Not every type pf cheese is totally carb free.
- ➤ If using the cream cheese melt or soft it, before stirring it into the batter.

- ➤ If using coconut flour, let the batter sit for 2-3 minutes to thicken up.

- ➤ It's better to use finely shredded cheese for the batter.

- ➤ To make your chaffle crispier sprinkle some extra cheese in the waffle iron before adding the batter.

- ➤ Do not open the waffle iron too early to check it. It should continue cooking until the chaffle is done and crisp. Let it cook for slightly longer for best results. It's best to cook most of the chaffle recipes for a minimum of 4 minutes, in general you will know the chaffle is ready when steam is no longer coming out of the sides.

- ➤ Mozzarella is always the best option because thanks to its mildness and it is not as greasy as many other cheese varieties.

➤ If you are using a nonstick saucepan to make your chaffles, grease and hot the pan before pouring the batter, then let it cook until golden brown and use a spatula to gently flip it.

Chaffle Maker

➤ There are many brands available, each with different cooking times and non-stick versions.

➤ Make sure that the surface is not too hot before you clean the waffle or chaffle maker.

➤ Use a damp cloth or paper towel for wiping away the crumbs.

➤ Soak up the excess oil drips on your grid plates.

➤ Wipe the exterior with the damp cloth or paper towel.

➤ Pour a few drops of cooking oil on the batter to remove the stubborn batter drips. Allow it to sit for a few minutes. Then wipe it away.

➤ Ensure that the waffle maker is completely dry before storing it.

- ➤ Always read the instruction manual before you use it for the first time.

- ➤ Just a light cooking oil coating is enough for nonstick waffle makers.

- ➤ Grease the grid with a little amount of oil if you see the waffles sticking.
- ➤ Never use metal or sharp tools to scrape off the batter or to remove the cooked waffles. You may end up scratching the surface and damaging it.

- ➤ Do not submerge your electric waffle maker in water.

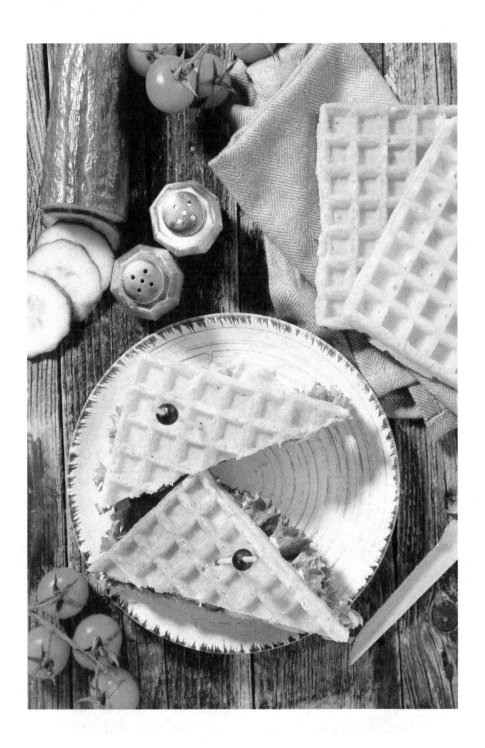

Chapter 1: Basic Chaffle Recipes

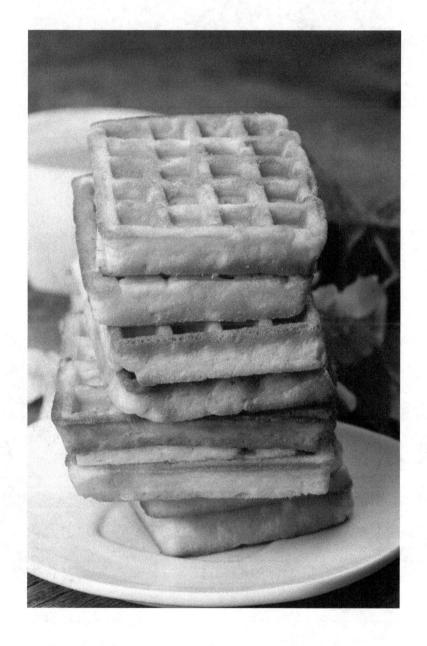

Egg-Free Psyllium Husk Chaffles

Preparation: 2 Minutes | Cooking: 4 Minutes | Servings: 1

Ingredients

- 1 ounce Mozzarella cheese, shredded
- 1 tablespoon cream cheese, softened
- 1 tablespoon psyllium husk powder

Directions

1. Preheat a waffle iron and then grease it.
2. In a blender, place all ingredients and pulse until a slightly crumbly mixture forms.
3. Place the mixture into preheated waffle iron and cook for about 4 minutes or until golden brown.
4. Serve warm.

Nutrition: Calories 208, Fat 13.5g, Carbohydrate 0.7g, Protein 8.2g, Sugars 0.6g

Simple Chaffle Toast

Cooking: 5 Minutes | Servings: 2

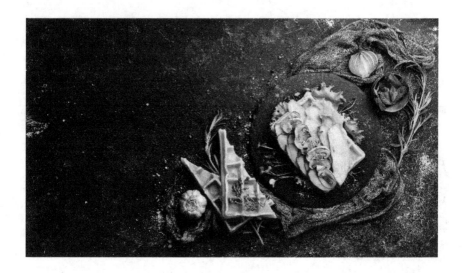

Ingredients

- 1 large egg
- 1/2 cup shredded cheddar cheese

Toppings:

- 1 egg
- 3-4 spinach leaves
- ¼ cup boil and shredded chicken

Directions

1. Preheat your square waffle maker on medium-high heat.

2. Mix together egg and cheese in a bowl and make two chaffles in a chaffle maker.
3. Once chaffle are cooked, carefully remove them from the maker.
4. Serve with spinach, boiled chicken, and fried egg.
5. Serve hot and enjoy!

Nutrition: Protein: 39% 99 kcal, Fat: % 153 kcal, Carbohydrates: 1% 3 kcal

Keto Sweet Bread Chaffle

Preparation: 10 minutes+ | Cooking: 3 minutes | Servings: 1

Ingredients

- 1 tbs almond flour
- 1 egg
- 1 tbs mayo we love this brand of mayo
- 1/8 tsp baking powder
- 1 tbs Allulose sweetener powdered
- 1/4 tsp cinnamon
- 1/8 tsp salt

Directions

1. Stir all ingredients: together. Let rest for 5 min.
2. Stir again.
3. Preheat the mini waffle iron
4. Put half of dough in mini waffle maker.
5. Cook 3 minutes.
6. Repeat. Let cool.

Nutrition: Calories: 199kcal, Carbohydrates: 3g, Protein: 7g, Fat: 18g, Saturated Fat: 3g , Cholesterol: 169mg, Sodium: 441mg, Potassium: 124mg, Fiber: 1g, Sugar: 1g, Vitamin A: 238IU, Calcium: 66mg

Parmesan Butter Chaffle

Preparation: 5 minutes | Cooking: 8 minutes | Servings: 2 chaffles

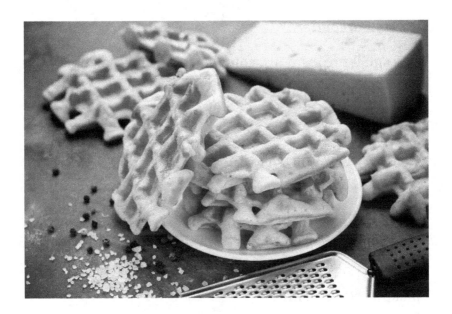

Ingredients

For the Chaffles

- 1 large egg, beaten
- ½ cup of mozzarella cheese, shredded
- 2 tbsp almond flour
- ¼ tsp baking powder

For Parmesan butter:

- 2 tbsp butter, softened

- 2 tbsp Parmesan cheese, shredded
- A pinch of salt and black pepper

Directions:

For Parmesan butter

1. In a small mixing bowl, combine all the ingredients and stir well. Set aside.

For chaffles:

1. Heat up the waffle maker.
2. Add all the chaffles ingredients to a small mixing bowl and combine well.
3. Pour half of the batter into the waffle maker and cook for 4 minutes until brown. Repeat with the rest of the batter to make another chaffle.
4. Let cool for 3 minutes to let chaffles get crispy.
5. Spread the chaffle with Parmesan butter.
6. Serve and enjoy!

Garlic Chaffles

Cooking: 5 Minutes | Servings: 4

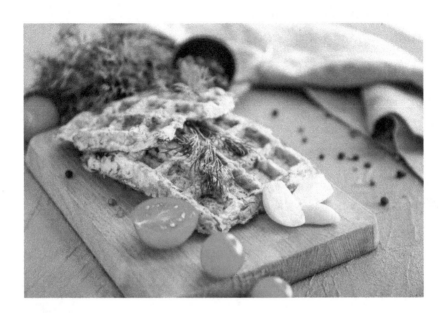

Ingredients

- 1/2 cup mozzarella cheese, shredded
- 1/3 cup cheddar cheese
- 1 large egg
- ½ tbsp. garlic powder
- 1/2 tsp Italian seasoning
- 1/4 tsp baking powder

Directions

1. Switch on your waffle maker and lightly grease your waffle maker with a brush.

2. Beat the egg with garlic powder, Italian seasoning and baking powder in a small mixing bowl.

3. Add mozzarella cheese and cheddar cheese tothe egg mixture and mix well.

4. Pour half of the chaffles batter into the middle of your waffle iron and close the lid.

5. Cook chaffles for about 2-3 minutes until crispy.

6. Once cooked, remove chaffles from the maker.

7. Sprinkle garlic powder on top and enjoy!

Nutrition: Calories 169, Total Fat 14.3g, Carbohydrate 4g, Fiber 4g, Protein 7.7g, Sugars 0.7g

Crispy Bagel Chaffles

Preparation: 10 min. | Cooking: 30 min. | Servings: 1

Ingredients

- 2 eggs
- ½ cup parmesan cheese
- 1 tsp bagel seasoning
- ½ cup mozzarella cheese
- 2 teaspoons almond flour

Directions

1. Turn on waffle maker to heat and oil it with cooking spray.
2. Evenly sprinkle half of cheeses to a griddle and let them melt. Then toast for 30 seconds and leave them wait for batter.
3. Whisk eggs, other half of cheeses, almond flour, and bagel seasoning in a small bowl. Pour batter into the waffle maker. Cook for 4 minutes.
4. Let cool for 2-3 minutes before serving.

Nutrition: Carbs: 6 g, Fat: 20 g, Protein: 21 g, Calories: 287

Peanut Butter Chaffle

Preparation: 15 min | Cooking: 10 min

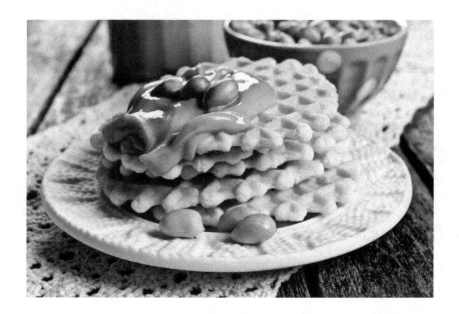

Ingredients

- 1 egg
- ½ cup of cheddar cheese
- 2 tablespoon of peanut butter
- Few drops of vanilla extract

Directions

1. To make deliciously tasting peanut butter chaffles. Take a grater and grate some cheddar cheese. Add one egg, cheddar cheese, 2 tablespoon of peanut butter, and a few

drops of vanilla extract. Beat these ingredients together until the batter is consistent enough.

2. Then sprinkle some shredded cheese as a base on the waffle maker. Pour the mixture on top of the waffle machine.

3. Sprinkle more cheese on top of the mixture and close the waffle machine. Ensure that the waffle is cooked thoroughly for about a few minutes until they are golden brown. Then remove it and enjoy your deliciously cooked chaffles.

Nutrition: 363 Calories, 29 g of Fat, 22 g of Protein, 4 g of Carbohydrates

Simple Chaffle

Preparation: 10 minutes | Cooking: 5 minutes | Servings: 4

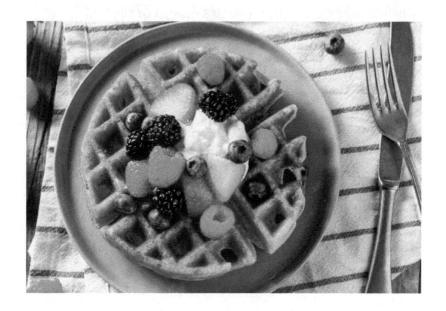

Ingredients

- 1 cup egg whites
- 1 cup cheddar cheese, shredded
- ¼ cup almond flour
- ¼ cup heavy cream
- 4 oz. raspberries
- 4 oz. strawberries.
- 1 oz. keto chocolate flakes
- 1 oz. feta cheese.

Directions

1. Preheat your square waffle maker and grease with cooking spray.
2. Beat egg white in a small bowl with flour.
3. Add shredded cheese to the egg whites and flour mixture and mix well.
4. Add cream and cheese to the egg mixture.
5. Pour Chaffles batter in a waffle maker and close the lid.
6. Cooking chaffles for about 4 minutes until crispy and brown.
7. Carefully remove chaffles from the maker.
8. Serve with berries, cheese, and chocolate on top.
9. Enjoy!

Nutrition: Calories: 254; Total Fat: 19g; Carbs: 11g; Net Carbs: 7g; Fiber: 4g; Protein: 11g

Sugar Free Sprinkles Chaffle

Preparation: 5 minutes | Cooking: 8 minutes | Servings: 2 chaffles

Ingredients

- 1 egg
- ½ cup shredded mozzarella cheese
- 1 tbsp almond flour
- 1 tbsp heavy whipping cream
- ½ tsp vanilla extract
- 1 tbsp sugar free sprinkles
- 2 tsp sweetener

Directions

1. Heat up the mini waffle maker.
2. Add all the ingredients to a small mixing bowl and combine well.
3. Pour half of the batter into the waffle maker and cook for 4 minutes. Repeat with the rest of the batter to make another chaffle.
4. Let cool for 3 minutes to let chaffles get crispy.
5. Top the chaffle with some sugar free whipped cream and a few sugar free sprinkles.
6. Serve and enjoy!

Egg-free Almond Flour Chaffles

Cooking: 10 Minutes | Servings: 2

Ingredients
- 2 tablespoons cream cheese, softened
- 1 cup mozzarella cheese, shredded
- 2 tablespoons almond flour
- 1 teaspoon organic baking powder

Directions

1. Preheat a mini waffle iron and then grease it.
2. In a medium bowl, place all ingredients: and with a fork, mix until well combined.
3. Place half of the mixture into preheated waffle iron and cook for about 4-5 minutes or until golden brown.
4. Repeat with the remaining mixture. Serve warm.

Nutrition: Calories: 77, Net Carb: 2.4g, Fat: 9.8g, Saturated Fat: 4g, Carbohydrates: 3.2g, Dietary Fiber: 0.8g, Sugar: 0.3g, Protein: 4.8g

Garlic Bread Chaffle

Cooking: 15 Minutes | Servings: 2

Ingredients

- 1 tbsp + 1tsp almond flour
- 1 egg
- 14 tsp baking powder
- 1/2 tsp garlic powder
- 1/8 tsp Italian seasoning
- 1 tbsp finely chopped cooked beef liver
- 1/4 tsp garlic salt
- 3 tsp unsalted butter (melted)
- 1/2 cup shredded mozzarella cheese
- 2 tbsp shredded parmesan cheese

Garnish:

- Chopped green onion

Directions

1. Preheat the oven to 375°F and line a baking sheet with parchment paper.
2. Plug the waffle maker to preheat it and spray it with non-stick spray.
3. In a mixing bowl, combine the almond flour, baking powder, Italian seasoning, garlic powder, beef liver and

cheese. Add the egg and mix until the ingredients are well combined.

4. Fill the waffle maker with appropriate amount of the batter and spread the batter to the edges of the waffle maker to cover all the holes on the waffle iron.

5. Close the lid of the waffle maker and cook for about 3 to 4 minutes or according to waffle maker's settings.

6. Meanwhile, whisk together the garlic salt and melted butter in a bowl.

7. After the cooking cycle, remove the chaffle from the waffle iron with a plastic or silicone utensil.

8. Repeat step 4, 5 and 7 until you have cooked all the batter into chaffles.

9. Brush the butter mixture over the face of each chaffle.

10. Top the chaffles with parmesan cheese and arrange them into the line baking sheet.

11. Place the sheet in the oven and bake for about 5 minutes or until the cheese melts.

12. Remove the bread chaffles from the oven and leave them to cool for a few minutes.

13. Serve warm and top with chopped green onions.

Nutrition: Fat 18g 23%, Carbohydrate 4.59 2%, Sugars 0.9g, Protein 12g

Chapter 2: Breakfast and Brunch Recipes

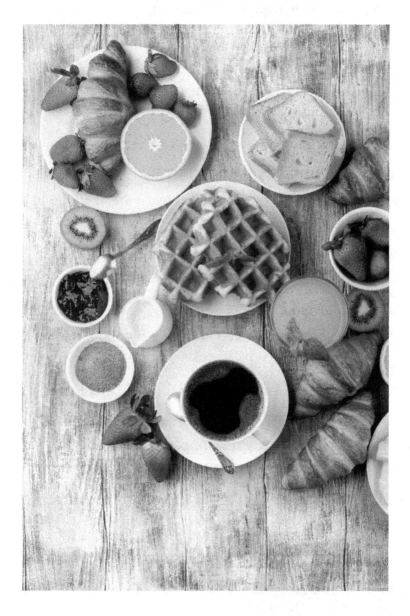

Breakfast Chaffle Sandwich

Preparation: 10 minutes | Cooking: 10 minutes | Servings: 1

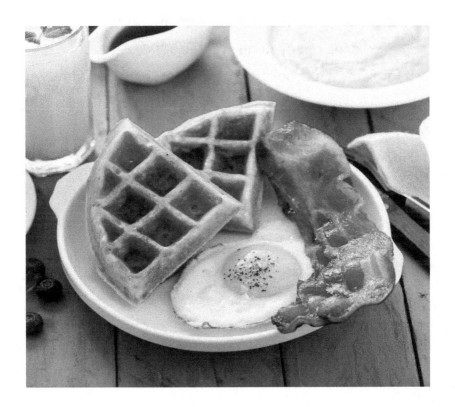

Ingredients

- 2 basics cooked chaffles (Choose a recipe you like from Chapter 1)
- Cooking spray
- 2 slices bacon
- 1 egg

Directions

1. Spray your pan with oil.
2. Place it over medium heat.
3. Cook the bacon until golden and crispy.
4. Put the bacon on top of one chaffle.
5. In the same pan, cook the egg without mixing until the yolk is set.
6. Add the egg on top of the bacon.
7. Top with another chaffle.

Italian Sausage Chaffles

Preparation: 5 minutes | Cooking: 8 minutes | Servings: 2

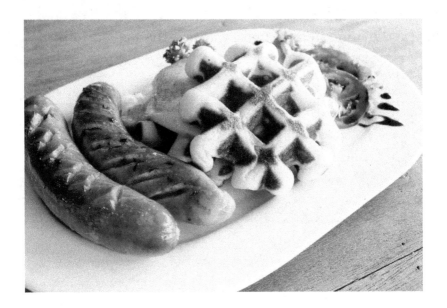

Ingredients

- 1 egg, beaten
- 1 cup cheddar cheese, shredded
- ¼ cup Parmesan cheese, grated
- 1 lb. Italian sausage, crumbled
- 2 teaspoons baking powder
- 1 cup almond flour

Directions

1. Preheat your waffle maker.
2. Mix all the ingredients in a bowl.

3. Pour half of the mixture into the waffle maker.
4. Cover and cook for 4 minutes.
5. Transfer to a plate.
6. Let cool to make it crispy.
7. Do the same steps to make the next chaffle.

Easter Morning Simple Chaffles

Cooking: 5 minutes | Servings: 2

Ingredients

- 1/2 cup egg whites
- 1 cup mozzarella cheese, melted

Directions

1. Switch on your square waffle maker. Spray with non-stick spray.
2. Beat egg whites with beater, until fluffy and white.
3. Add cheese and mix well.
4. Pour batter in a waffle maker.
5. Close the maker and cook for about 3 minutes.
6. Repeat with the remaining batter.
7. Remove chaffles from the maker.
8. Serve hot and enjoy!

Nutrition: Protein: 36% 42 kcal, Fat: 60% 71kcal, Carbohydrates: 4% 5 kcal

Keto Chaffle Cheddar

Preparation: 5 minutes | Cooking: 3-5 minutes | Servings: 1

Ingredients

- 1 Egg
- ⅓ Cup Shredded cheddar cheese
- 1 ½ Tbsp. Heavy whipping cream
- 1 Tbsp. Almond flour
- Salt and pepper to taste
- Mini waffle iron

Directions

1. Heat up your mini waffle iron.
2. Mix together the ingredients in a mixing bowl until well combined.
3. Place half of the batter mixture into the mini waffle maker, and cook for 3-5 minutes, or until the chaffle is done to your liking.
4. Remove the first chaffle from the mini waffle iron, and place the other half of the batter in to cook.

Cinnamon Roll Chaffle

Cooking: 9 Minutes | Servings: 3

Ingredients

- 1 egg (beaten)
- 1/2 cup shredded mozzarella cheese
- 1 tsp cinnamon
- 1 tsp sugar free maple syrup
- 1/4 tsp baking powder
- 1 tbsp almond flour
- 1/2 tsp vanilla extract

Topping:

- 2 tsp granulated swerve
- 1 tbsp heavy cream
- 4 tbsp cream cheese

Directions:

1. Plug the waffle maker to preheat it and spray it with a non-stick spray.
2. In a mixing bowl, whisk together the egg, maple syrup and vanilla extract.
3. In another mixing bowl, combine the cinnamon, almond flour, baking powder and mozzarella cheese. Pour in the

egg mixture into the flour mixture and mix until the ingredients are well combined.

4. Pour in an appropriate amount of the batter into the waffle maker and spread out the batter to the edges to cover all the holes on the waffle maker.
5. Close the waffle maker and bake for about 3 minute or according to your waffle maker's settings.
6. After the cooking cycle, use a silicone or plastic utensil to remove the chaffle from the waffle maker.
7. Repeat step 5 to 7 until you have cooked all the batter into chaffles.
8. For the TOPPING, combine the cream cheese, swerve and heavy cream in a microwave safe dish.
9. Place the dish in a microwave and microwave on high until the mixture is melted and smooth. Stir every 15 seconds.
10. Top the chaffles with the cream mixture and enjoy.

Nutrition: Fat 9.99 13%, Carbohydrate 3.8g 1%, Sugars 0.3g, Protein 4.8g

Avocado Chaffles

Cooking: 5 Minutes | Servings: 2

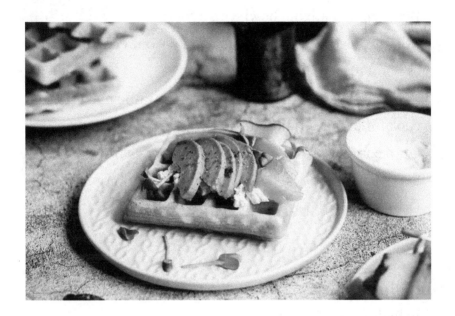

Ingredients

- 1 large egg
- 1/2 cup finely shredded mozzarella
- 1/8 cup avocado mash
- 1 tbsp. coconut cream

Topping:

- 2 oz. smoked salmon
- 1 Avocado thinly sliced

Directions:

1. Switch on your square waffle maker and grease with cooking spray.
2. Beat egg in a mixing bowl with a fork.
3. Add the cheese, avocado mash and coconut cream to the egg and mix well.
4. Pour chaffle mixture in the preheated waffle maker and cook for about 2-3 minutes.
5. Once chaffles are cooked, carefully remove from the maker.
6. Serve with an avocado slice and smoked salmon.
7. Drizzle ground pepper on top.
8. Enjoy!

Nutrition: Protein: 23% kcal, Fat: 67% 266 kcal, Carbohydrates: 11% 42 kcal

Bacon Chaffles With Herb Dip

Cooking: 10 Minutes | Servings: 2

Ingredients

Chaffle:

- 1 organic egg, beaten
- 1/2 cup Swiss/Gruyere cheese blend, shredded
- 2 tablespoons cooked bacon pieces
- 1 tablespoon jalapeno pepper, chopped

Dip:

- 1/4 cup heavy cream
- 1/4 teaspoon fresh dill, minced
- Pinch of ground black pepper

Directions

1. Preheat a mini waffle iron and then grease it.
2. In a medium bowl, put all Ingredients and mix well.
3. Place half of the mixture into preheated waffle iron and cook for about 5 minutes.
4. Repeat with the remaining mixture.
5. Meanwhile, for dip: in a bowl, mix together the cream and stevia.
6. Serve warm chaffles alongside the dip.

Nutrition: Calories 210, Net Carbs 2.2 g, Total Fat 13 g, Saturated Fat 9.7 g, Cholesterol 132 mg, Sodium 164 mg, Total Carbs 2.3 g, Fiber 0.1 g, Sugar 0.7 g, Protein n.g g

Jalapeno Bacon Swiss Chaffle

Preparation: 18 minutes   Cooking: 12 minutes | Servings: 2

Ingredients

- Shredded Swiss cheese: ½ cup
- Fresh jalapenos (diced): 1 tablespoon
- Bacon piece: 2 tablespoons
- Egg: 1

Directions

1. First, preheat and grease the waffle maker.
2. Using a pan, cooking the bacon pieces, put off the heat and shred the cheese and egg.
3. Add in the diced fresh jalapenos and mix evenly.
4. Heat the waffle makers to get the mixture into a crispy form.
5. Repeat the process for the remaining mixture.
6. Serve the dish to enjoy.

Nutrition: Calories 329, Fat 16, Carbs 10, Protein 23

Chaffle Tacos

Preparation: 5 minutes | Cooking: 8 Minutes | Servings: 2

Ingredients

- 1 egg white
- 1/4 cup Monterey jack cheese, shredded (packed tightly)
- 1/4 cup sharp cheddar cheese, shredded (packed tightly)
- 3/4 tsp. water
- 1 tsp. coconut flour
- 1/4 tsp. baking powder
- 1/8 tsp. chili powder
- Pinch of salt

Directions

1. Plug the Dash Mini Waffle Maker in the wall and grease lightly once it is hot.
2. Combine all of the ingredients in a bowl and stir to combine.
3. Spoon out 1/2 of the batter on the waffle maker and close lid. Set a timer for 4 minutes and do not lift the lid until the cooking time is complete. If you do, it will look like the taco chaffle shell isn't set up properly, but it will. You have to let it cooking the entire 4 minutes before lifting the lid.

4. Remove the taco chaffle shell from the waffle iron and set aside. Repeat the same steps above with the rest of the chaffle batter.
5. Turn over a muffin pan and set the taco chaffle shells between the cups to form a taco shell. Allow the setting for a few minutes.
6. Enjoy this delicious keto crispy taco chaffle shell with your favorite toppings.

Nutrition: Calories 174, Fat 15, Carbs 5, Protein 7

Chatper 3: Savory Recipes

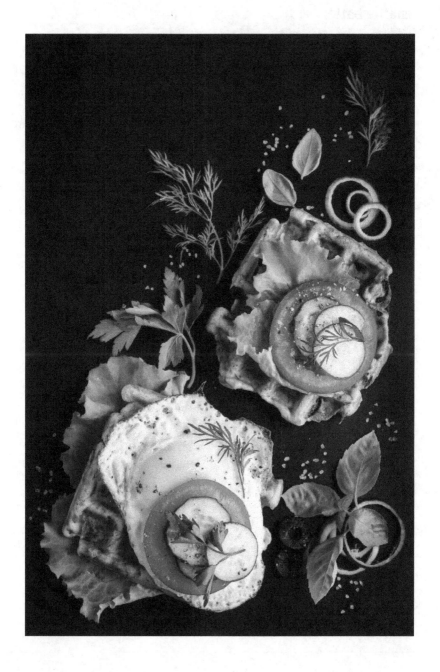

Chicken Bacon Chaffle

Preparation: 5 min. | Cooking: 5 min. | Servings: 2

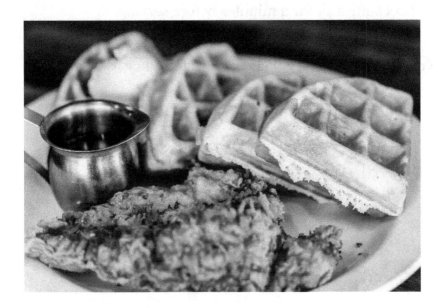

Ingredients

- 1 egg
- ⅓ cup cooked chicken, diced
- 1 piece of bacon, cooked and crumbled
- ⅓ cup shredded cheddar jack cheese
- 1 tsp powdered ranch dressing

Directions

1. Turn on waffle maker to heat and oil it with cooking spray. Mix egg, dressing, and Monterey cheese in a small bowl. Add bacon and chicken.

2. Add half of the batter to the waffle maker and cook for 3-4 minutes. Remove and cook remaining batter to make a second chaffle.

3. Let chaffles sit for 2 minutes before serving.

Nutrition: Carbs: 2 g, Fat: 14 g, Protein: 16 g, Calories: 200

Spiced Pumpkin Chaffles

Cooking: 8 Minutes | Servings: 2

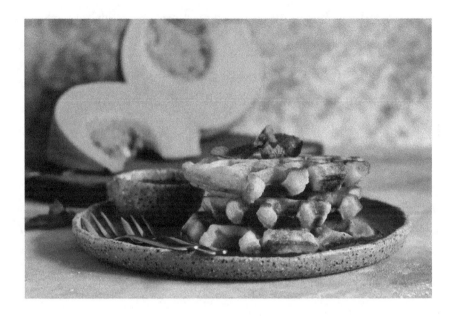

Ingredients

- 1 organic egg, beaten
- ½ cup Mozzarella cheese, shredded
- 1 tablespoon sugar-free canned solid pumpkin
- ¼ teaspoon ground cinnamon
- Pinch of ground cloves
- Pinch of ground nutmeg
- Pinch of ground ginger

Directions

1. Preheat a mini waffle iron and then grease it.
2. In a medium bowl, place all ingredients and with a fork, mix until well combined.
3. Place half of the mixture into preheated waffle iron and cook for about 4 minutes or until golden brown.
4. Repeat with the remaining mixture.
5. Serve warm.

Nutrition: Calories: 98, Fat: 3.5g, Carbohydrates: 1.4g, Sugar: 0.5g, Protein: 4.9g

Colby Jack Chaffles

Cooking: 6 Minutes | Servings: 1

Ingredients

- 2 ounces colby jack cheese, sliced thinly in triangles
- 1 large organic egg, beaten

Directions

1. Preheat a waffle iron and then grease it.
2. Arrange 1 thin layer of cheese slices in the bottom of preheated waffle iron.
3. Place the beaten egg on top of the cheese.
4. Now, arrange another layer of cheese slices on top to cover evenly.
5. Cook for about 6 minutes.
6. Serve warm.

Nutrition: Calories 292, Fat 23 g, Carbs 2.4 g, Sugar 0.4 g, Protein 18.3 g

Ham and Jalapenos Chaffle

Cooking: 9 Minutes | Servings: 3

Ingredients

- 2 lbs cheddar cheese, finely grated
- 2 large eggs
- ½ jalapeno pepper, finely grated
- 2 ounces ham steak
- 1 medium scallion
- 2 tsp coconut flour

Directions

1. Spray your waffle iron with cooking spray and heat for 3 minutes.
2. Pour 1/4 of the batter mixture into the waffle iron.
3. Cook for 3 minutes, until crispy around the edges.
4. Remove the waffles from the heat and repeat until all the batter is finished.
5. Once done, allow them to cool to room temperature and enjoy.
6. Shred the cheddar cheese using a fine grater.
7. Deseed the jalapeno and grate using the same grater.
8. Finely chop the scallion and ham.

Nutrition: Calories 120 ; Fat: 10 g ; Carbs: 2 g ; Protein: 12

Bbq Chicken Chaffles

Cooking: 8 Minutes | Servings: 2

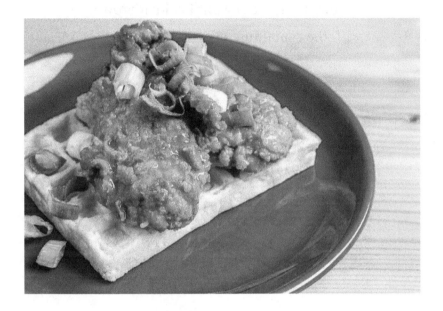

Ingredients

- 1. 1/3 cups grass-fed cooked chicken, chopped
- ½ cup Cheddar cheese, shredded
- 1 tablespoon sugar-free BBQ sauce
- 1 organic egg, beaten
- 1 tablespoon almond flour

Directions

1. Preheat a mini waffle iron and then grease it.

2. In a bowl, place all ingredients and mix until well combined.
3. Place half of the mixture into preheated waffle iron and cook for about 4 minutes or until golden brown.
4. Repeat with the remaining mixture.
5. Serve warm.

Nutrition: Calories: 320, Fat: 16.3g, Carbohydrates: 4g, Sugar: 2g, Protein: 36.9g

Avocado Chaffle

Cooking: 10 Minutes | Servings: 2

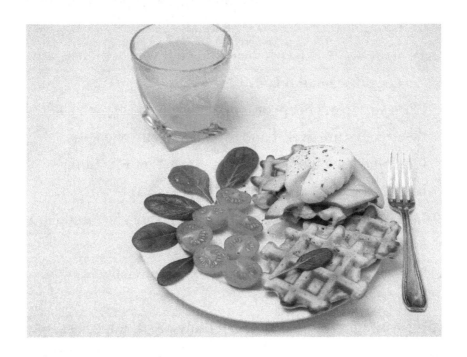

Ingredients

- ½ avocado, sliced
- ½ tsp lemon juice
- ⅛ tsp salt
- ⅛ tsp black pepper
- 1 egg
- ½ cup shredded cheese
- ¼ crumbled feta cheese
- 1 cherry tomato, halved

Directions

1. Mash together avocado, lemon juice, salt, and pepper until well-combined.

2. Turn on waffle maker to heat and oil it with cooking spray.

3. Beat egg in a small mixing bowl.

4. Place ⅛ cup of cheese on waffle maker, then spread half of the egg mixture over it and top with ⅛ cup of cheese.

5. Close and cook for 3-4 minutes. Repeat for remaining batter.

6. Let chaffles cool for 3-4 minutes, then spread avocado mix on top of each.

7. Top with crumbled feta and cherry tomato halves.

Nutrition: Carbs: 5 g ; Fat: 19 g ;Protein: 7 g ;Calories: 232

Zucchini & Onion Chaffles

Cooking: 16 Minutes | Servings: 4

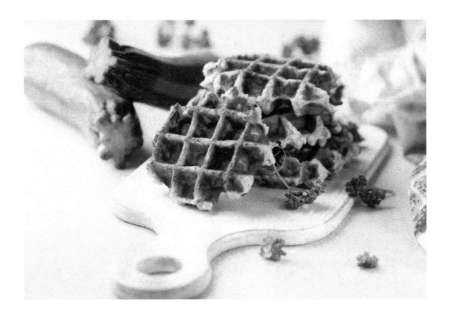

Ingredients

- 2 cups zucchini, grated and squeezed
- ½ cup onion, grated and squeezed
- 2 organic eggs
- ½ cup Mozzarella cheese, shredded
- ½ cup Parmesan cheese, grated

Directions

1. Preheat a waffle iron and then grease it.

2. In a medium bowl, place all ingredients and, mix until well combined.
3. Place ¼ of the mixture into preheated waffle iron and cook for about 4 minutes or until golden brown.
4. Repeat with the remaining mixture.
5. Serve warm.

Nutrition: Calories: 92, Fat: 5.3g, Carbohydrates: 3.5g, Sugar: 1.8g, Protein: 8.6g

Chaffle Cuban Sandwich

Preparation: 10 min. | Cooking: 10 min. | Servings: 1

Ingredients

- 1 large egg
- 1 Tbsp almond flour
- 1 Tbsp full-fat Greek yogurt
- ⅛ tsp baking powder
- ¼ cup shredded Swiss cheese

For the filling:

- 3 oz roast pork
- 2 oz deli ham
- 1 slice Swiss cheese
- 3-5 sliced pickle chips
- ½ Tbsp Dijon mustard

Directions

1. Turn on waffle maker to heat and oil it with cooking spray.
2. Beat egg, yogurt, almond flour, and baking powder in a bowl.
3. Sprinkle ¼ Swiss cheese on hot waffle maker. Top with half of the egg mixture, then add ¼ of the cheese on top. Close and cook for 3-5 minutes, until golden brown and crispy.
4. Repeat with remaining batter.

5. Layer pork, ham, and cheese slice in a small microwaveable bowl. Microwave for 50 seconds, until cheese melts.

6. Spread the inside of chaffle with mustard and top with pickles. Invert bowl onto chaffle top so that cheese is touching pickles. Place bottom chaffle onto pork and serve.

Nutrition: Carbs: 4 g, Fat: 46 g, Protein: 33 g, Calories: 522

3 Cheeses Herbed Chaffles

Cooking: 12 Minutes | Servings: 4

Ingredients

- 4 tablespoons almond flour
- 1 tablespoon coconut flour
- 1 teaspoon mixed dried herbs
- ½ teaspoon organic baking powder
- ¼ teaspoon garlic powder
- ¼ teaspoon onion powder
- Salt and freshly ground black pepper, to taste
- ¼ cup cream cheese, softened
- 3 large organic eggs
- ½ cup Cheddar cheese, grated
- 1/3 cup Parmesan cheese, grated

Directions

1. Preheat a waffle iron and then grease it.
2. In a bowl, mix together the flours, dried herbs, baking powder and seasoning and mix well.
3. In a separate bowl, put cream cheese and eggs and beat until well combined.
4. Add the flour mixture, cheddar and Parmesan cheese and mix until well combined.

5. Place the desired amount of the mixture into preheated waffle iron and cook for about 2-3 minutes or until golden brown.
6. Repeat with the remaining mixture.
7. Serve warm

Nutrition: Calories: 240, Fat: 19g, Carbohydrates: 4g, Sugar: 0.7g, Protein: 12.3g

Bagel Seasoning Chaffles

Cooking: 20 Minutes | Servings: 4

Ingredients

- 1 large organic egg
- 1 cup Mozzarella cheese, shredded
- 1 tablespoon almond flour
- 1 teaspoon organic baking powder
- 2 teaspoons bagel seasoning
- ¼ teaspoon garlic powder
- ¼ teaspoon onion powder

Directions

1. Preheat a mini waffle iron and then grease it.
2. In a medium bowl, place all ingredients and with a fork, mix until well combined.
3. Place ¼ of the mixture into preheated waffle iron and cook for about 4 minutes or until golden brown.
4. Repeat with the remaining mixture.
5. Serve warm.

Nutrition: Calories: 73, Fat: 5.5g, Carbohydrates: 2.3g, Sugar: 0.9g, Protein: 3.7g

Grilled Cheese Chaffle

Cooking: 10 Minutes | Servings: 1

Ingredients

- 1 large egg
- ½ cup mozzarella cheese
- 2 slices yellow American cheese
- 2-3 slices cooked bacon, cut in half
- 1 tsp butter
- ½ tsp baking powder

Directions

1. Turn on waffle maker to heat and oil it with cooking spray.
2. Beat egg in a bowl.
3. Add mozzarella, and baking powder.
4. Pour half of the mix into the waffle maker and cook for minutes.
5. Remove and repeat to make the second chaffle.
6. Layer bacon and cheese slices in between two chaffles.
7. Melt butter in a skillet and add chaffle sandwich to the pan. Fry on each side for 2-3 minutes covered, until cheese has melted.
8. Slice in half on a plate and serve.

Nutrition: Carbs: 4 g; Fat: 18 g ; Protein: 7 g ; Calories: 233

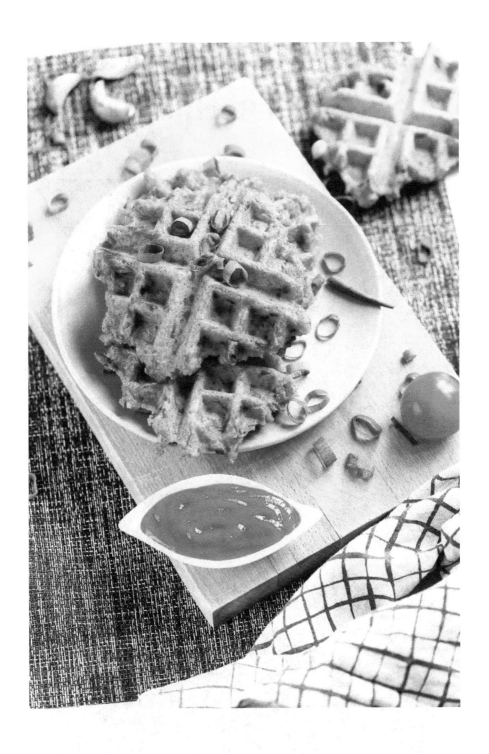

Chapter 4: Sandwich and Pizza Recipes

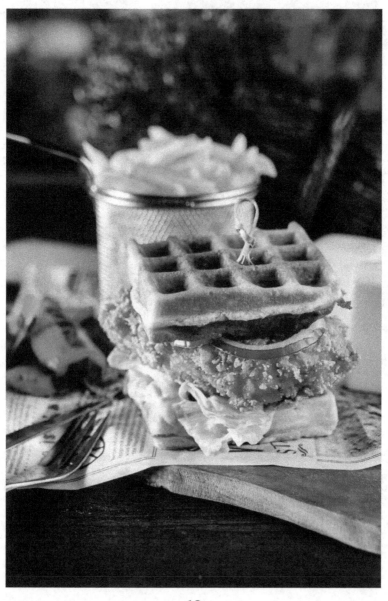

Pumpkin Pizza Chaffle

Preparation: 5 minutes | Cooking: 13 minutes | Servings: 2 chaffles

Ingredients

For chaffles:

- ½ cup shredded mozzarella cheese
- 1 tbsp almond flour
- ½ tsp baking powder
- 1 egg, beaten
- A pinch of salt and pepper

For topping:

- 2 tbsp low carb pasta sauce
- 2 tbsp mozzarella cheese, shredded
- 1 tbsp baked pumpkin, diced
- 1 tsp dried or fresh rosemary

Directions

1. Heat up the waffle maker.
2. Add all the chaffle ingredients to a small mixing bowl and combine well.
3. Pour down half of the batter into the waffle maker and cook for about 4 minutes until golden brown color. Repeat now with the rest of the batter to make another chaffle.

4. Once both chaffles are cooked, place them on the baking sheet of the toaster oven.
5. Put 1 tbsp of low carb pasta sauce on top of each chaffle.
6. Sprinkle 1 tbsp of shredded mozzarella cheese on top of each one.
7. Top with diced pumpkin and sprinkle with rosemary.
8. Bake it at 350° in the toaster oven for about 2-3 minutes, until the cheese is melted.
9. Serve and enjoy!

Rosemary Bacon Pizza Chaffle

Preparation: 5 minutes | Cooking: 13 minutes | Servings: 2 chaffles

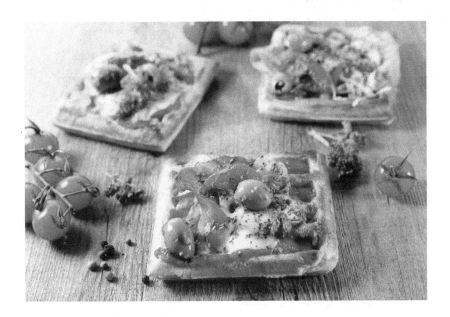

Ingredients

For chaffles:

- ½ cup shredded mozzarella cheese
- 1 tbsp almond flour
- ½ tsp baking powder
- 1 egg, beaten
- A pinch of salt and pepper

For topping:

- 2 tbsp low carb pasta sauce
- 2 tbsp mozzarella cheese, shredded
- 1 tbsp bacon, diced
- 1 tsp dried or fresh rosemary

Directions

1. Heat up the waffle maker.
2. Add all the chaffle ingredients to a small mixing bowl and combine well.
3. Pour down half of the batter into the waffle maker and cook for about 4 minutes until golden brown color. Repeat now with the rest of the batter to make another chaffle.
4. Once both chaffles are cooked, place them on the baking sheet of the toaster oven.
5. Put 1 tbsp of low carb pasta sauce on top of each chaffle.
6. Sprinkle 1 tbsp of shredded mozzarella cheese on top of each one.
7. Top with diced bacon and sprinkle with rosemary.
8. Bake it at 350° in the toaster oven for about 2-3 minutes, until the cheese is melted.
9. Serve and enjoy!

Ham and Mushrooms Pizza Chaffle

Preparation: 5 minutes | Cooking: 10 minutes | Servings: 2 chaffles

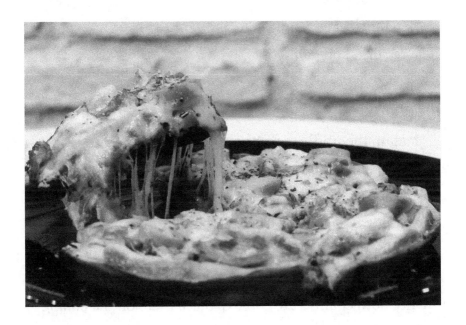

Ingredients

For chaffles:

- ½ cup shredded mozzarella cheese
- 1 tbsp almond flour
- ½ tsp baking powder
- 1 egg, beaten
- A pinch of salt

For topping:

- 2 tbsp low carb pasta sauce
- 2 tbsp mozzarella cheese, shredded
- 2 slices of ham
- 2 tsp mushrooms, minced
- ¼ tsp dried oregano

Directions

1. Heat up the waffle maker.
2. Add all the chaffle ingredients to a small mixing bowl and combine well.
3. Pour down half of the batter into the waffle maker and cook for about 4 minutes until golden brown color. Repeat with the rest of the batter to make another chaffle.
4. Once both chaffles are cooked, place them on the baking sheet of the toaster oven.
5. Put 1 tbsp of low carb pasta sauce on the top of each chaffle.
6. Sprinkle 1 tbsp of shredded mozzarella cheese on top of each one.
7. Top with a slice of ham and mushrooms. Sprinkle with oregano.
8. Bake it at 350° in the toaster oven for about 2 minutes, until the cheese is melted.
9. Serve and enjoy!

Cauliflower Pizza Chaffle

Preparation: 5 minutes | Cooking: 13 minutes | Servings: 2 pizza chaffles

Ingredients

For chaffles:

- ½ cup shredded mozzarella cheese
- 1 tbsp almond flour
- ½ tsp baking powder
- 1 egg, beaten
- 1 tbsp grated cauliflower

For topping:

- 2 tbsp low carb pasta sauce
- 2 tbsp mozzarella cheese, shredded
- ½ tbsp green bell pepper, thinly sliced
- 1 tsp dried oregano

Directions

1. Heat up the waffle maker.
2. Add all the chaffle ingredients to a small mixing bowl and combine well.
3. Pour down half of the batter into the waffle maker and cook for about 4 minutes. Now, repeat with the rest of the batter to make another pizza chaffle.

4. Once both chaffles are cooked, place them on the baking sheet of the oven.

5. Put 1 tbsp of low carb pasta sauce on top of each chaffle.

6. Sprinkle now 1 tablespoon of shredded mozzarella cheese on top of each one.

7. Top chaffle with green bell peppers and oregano.

8. Bake at 350° in the oven for about 5 minutes, until the cheese is melted.

9. Serve and enjoy!

Chicken Sandwich Chaffle

Preparation: 6 minutes. | Cooking: 8 Minutes | Servings: 2

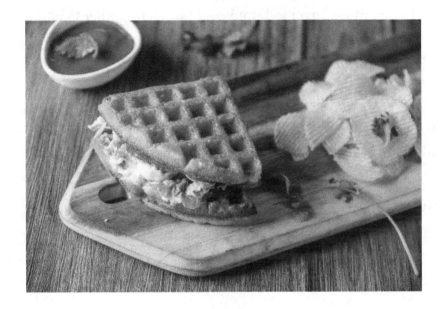

Ingredients

Chaffles:

- 1 large organic egg, beaten
- ½ cup cheddar cheese, shredded
- Pinch of salt and ground black pepper

Filling:

- 1 (6-ounce) cooked chicken breast, halved
- 2 lettuce leaves
- ¼ of small onion, sliced
- 1 small tomato, sliced

Directions

1. Preheat a mini waffle iron and then grease it.
2. For chaffles: In a medium bowl, put all ingredients and with a fork, mix until well combined. Place down half of the mixture into preheated waffle iron and cook for about 3–4 minutes.
3. Repeat with the remaining mixture.
4. Serve each chaffle with filling ingredients.

Nutrition: Calories: 194, Fat: 3.8g, Carbs: 29.0g, Protein: 10.9g, Fiber: 9.4g

Bacon and Cheese Chaffle Sandwich

Preparation: 30 mins | Cooking: 5 mins

Ingredients

- 1 egg
- ½ cup of shredded mozzarella cheese
- 2 Tablespoon of coconut flour
- ½ tsp of baking powder
- 1 teaspoon of Italian herbs
- 2 tablespoon of almond oil
- 1 slice of cheddar cheese
- 2 bacon strips

Directions

1. Start with a simple chaffle base. Mix in a bowl shredded mozzarella cheese, coconut flour, baking powder, Italian herbs, and an egg.
2. Whisk this mixture well. Then take a waffle machine and preheat it to around medium heat.
3. Once it is preheated, sprinkle some cheese on the waffle machine. Add the mixture on top of the cheese base and top it off with more cheese.
4. Let this cook in the machine for 4 minutes until the color changes to a golden brown.

5. Then turn the heat below a pan. Then add almond oil in the pan, cook the bacon strips in the oil. Take them out once they are fried.
6. Now it is time for the assembly of the sandwich. Add your bacon and cheese to the sandwich and enjoy it.

Nutrition: Calories 449, Fat 30g, Protein 24g, Carbohydrates 2.2g

Peanut Butter Sandwich Chaffle

Preparation: 15 minutes | Servings: 1

Ingredients

For chaffle:

- 1 egg, lightly beaten
- 1/2 cup mozzarella cheese, shredded
- 1/4 tsp espresso powder
- 1 tbsp unsweetened chocolate chips
- 1 tbsp Swerve
- 2 tbsp unsweetened cocoa powder

For filling:

- 1 tbsp butter, softened
- 2 tbsp Swerve
- 3 tbsp creamy peanut butter

Directions

1. Preheat your waffle maker.
2. In a bowl, whisk together egg, espresso powder, chocolate chips, Swerve, and cocoa powder.
3. Add mozzarella cheese and stir well.
4. Spray waffle maker with cooking spray.

5. Pour down 1/2 of the batter in the hot waffle maker and cook for 3-4 minutes or until golden brown. Repeat with the remaining batter.
6. For filling: In a tiny bowl, stir together butter, Swerve, and peanut butter until smooth.
7. Once chaffles is cool, then spread filling mixture between two chaffle and place in the fridge for 10 minutes.
8. Cut chaffle sandwich in half and serve.

Berry Sauce and Sandwich Chaffles

Preparation: 6 minutes | Cooking: 8 Minutes | Servings: 2

Ingredients

Filling:

- 3 ounces frozen mixed berries, thawed with the juice
- 1 tablespoon erythritol
- 1 tablespoon water
- ¼ tablespoon fresh lemon juice
- 2 teaspoons cream

Chaffles:

- 1 large organic egg, beaten
- ½ cup cheddar cheese, shredded
- 2 tablespoons almond flour

Directions

1. For berry sauce: in a pan, add the berries, erythritol, water and lemon juice over medium heat and cook for about 8– minutes, pressing with the spoon occasionally.
2. Remove the pan of sauce from heat and set aside to cool before serving.
3. Preheat a mini waffle iron and then grease it.

4. In a bowl, add the egg, cheddar cheese and almond flour and beat until well combined. Place down half of the mixture into preheated waffle iron and cook for about 3–5 min.
5. Repeat with the remaining mixture.
6. Serve each chaffle with cream and berry sauce.

Nutrition: Calories: 548, Fat: 20.7g, Protein: 46g

Pork Sandwich Chaffle

Preparation: 6 minutes | Cooking: 16 Minutes | Servings: 4

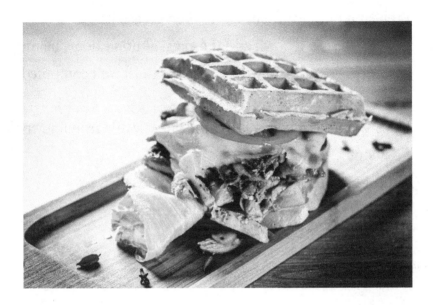

Ingredients

Chaffles:

- 2 large organic eggs
- ¼ cup superfine blanched almond flour
- ¾ teaspoon organic baking powder
- ½ teaspoon garlic powder
- 1 cup cheddar cheese, shredded

Filling:

- 12 ounces cooked pork, cut into slices
- 1 tomato, sliced

- 4 lettuce leaves

Directions

1. Preheat a mini waffle iron and then grease it.
2. For chaffles: in a bowl, add the eggs, almond flour, baking powder, and garlic powder, and beat until well combined.
3. Add the cheese and stir to combine.
4. Place ¼ of the mixture into preheated waffle iron and cook for about 3–minutes.
5. Repeat with the remaining mixture.
6. Serve each chaffle with filling ingredients.

Nutrition: Calories: 67, Fat: 8g, Protein: 3g, Sugar: 0g

Tomato Sandwich Chaffle

Preparation: 6 minutes | Cooking: 6 Minutes | Servings: 2

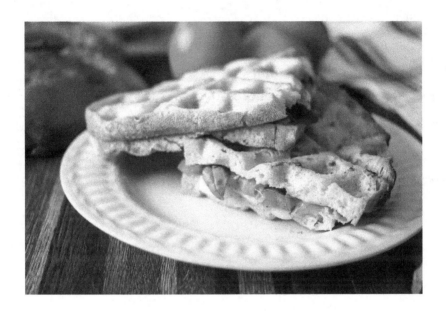

Ingredients

Chaffles:

- 1 large organic egg, beaten
- ½ cup Colby jack cheese, shredded finely
- 1/8 teaspoon organic vanilla extract

Filling:

- 1 small tomato, sliced
- 2 teaspoons fresh basil leaves

Directions

1. Preheat a mini waffle iron and then grease it.
2. For chaffles: in a small bowl, place all the ingredients and stir to combine.
3. Place down half of the mixture into preheated waffle iron and cook for about minutes.
4. Repeat with the remaining mixture.
5. Serve each chaffle with tomato slices and basil leaves.

Nutrition: Calories: 285, Fat: 20.5g, Protein: 8.6g

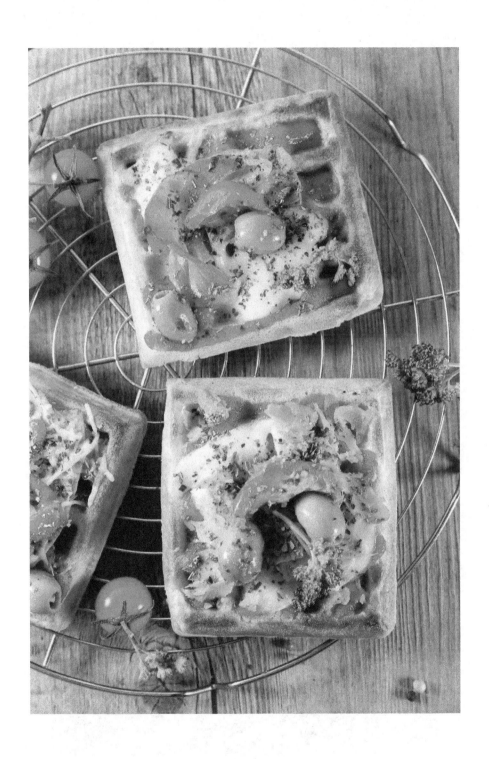

Chapter 5: Sweets and Desserts

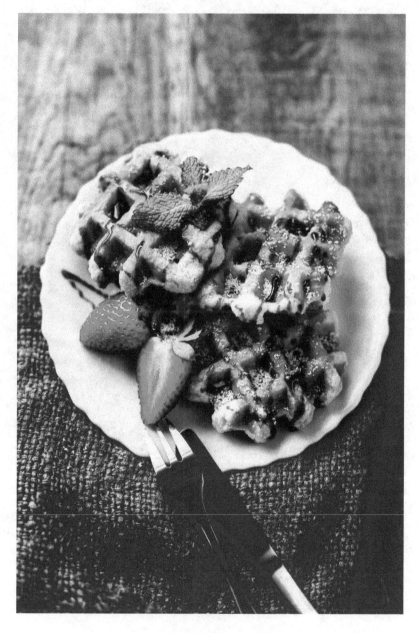

Choco Coco Chaffle

Preparation: 5 minutes | Cooking: 8 minutes | Servings: 2 chaffles

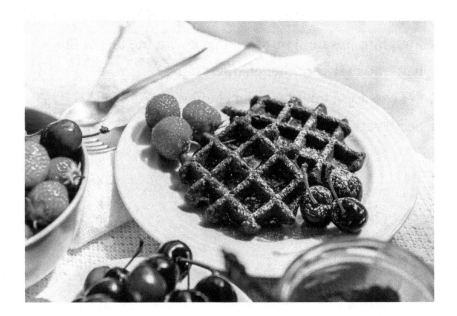

Ingredients

- 1 egg, beaten
- ½ cup mozzarella cheese, grated
- 1 tsp coconut flour
- 1 tsp water
- ¼ tsp baking powder
- 2 tbsp chocolate chips, unsweetened

Directions

1. Heat up the waffle maker.
2. Now, add all the ingredients to a small mixing bowl and stir until well combined.
3. Now, pour half of the batter into the waffle maker and cook for 4 minutes until brown. Repeat with the rest of the batter to make another chaffle.
4. Let cool for 3 minutes to let chaffles get crispy.
5. Serve with cocoa powder and enjoy!

Coconut Chaffle with Berries

Preparation: 5 minutes | Cooking: 16 minutes | Servings: 4 chaffles

Ingredients

For Chaffles

- 2 tbsp softened cream cheese
- 2 eggs, beaten
- 1 cup mozzarella cheese, shredded
- 4 tbsp coconut flour
- 1 tsp baking powder
- 1 tbsp butter, melted
- 2 tsp vanilla extract
- 1 tbsp sweetener

For Topping:

- 4 tsp sweetener
- 4 tbsp fresh blackberries
- 4 tbsp fresh raspberries
- 4 tbsp fresh blueberries

Directions

1. Heat up the waffle maker.

2. Add all the chaffles ingredients to a small mixing bowl and stir until well combined.

3. Pour ¼ of the batter into your waffle maker and cook for 4 minutes. Then cook the remaining batter to make the other chaffles.

4. Top the chaffles with berries and sprinkle with sweetener.

5. Serve and enjoy!

Cereals & Walnuts Chaffle

Preparation: 5 minutes | Cooking: 8 minutes | Servings: 2 chaffles

Ingredients

- 1 large egg, beaten
- 2 tbsp almond flour
- 1 tbsp cereals, minced
- ¼ tsp baking powder
- 1 tbsp butter, melted
- 1 tbsp cream cheese, softened
- ¼ tsp vanilla powder
- 1 tbsp sweetener
- ½ tbsp walnuts, chopped

Directions

1. Heat up the waffle maker.
2. Now, add all the ingredients to a small mixing bowl and stir until well combined.
3. Now, pour half of the batter into the waffle maker and cook for 4 minutes. Now, repeat with the rest of the batter to make another chaffle.
4. Serve with keto caramel sauce and enjoy!

Eggnog Chaffle

Preparation: 5 minutes | Cooking: 8 minutes | Servings: 2 chaffles

Ingredients

- 1 egg, beaten
- 2 tbsp cream cheese, softened
- 2 tsp sweetener
- 2 tbsp coconut flour
- ½ tsp baking powder
- ¼ cup keto eggnog
- A pinch of nutmeg

Directions

1. Heat up the waffle maker.
2. Now, add all the ingredients to a small mixing bowl and stir until well combined.
3. Now, pour half of the batter into the waffle maker and cook for 4 minutes. Now, repeat with the rest of the batter to make another chaffle.
4. Let cool for 3 minutes to let chaffles get crispy.
5. Serve and enjoy!

Chocolate Chaffle with Eggnog Topping

Preparation: 5 minutes | Cooking: 8 minutes | Servings: 2 chaffles

Ingredients

For Chaffles

- ½ cup shredded mozzarella cheese
- 1 tbsp almond flour
- 1 egg, beaten
- ¼ tsp cinnamon
- ½ tbsp sweetener
- 2 tbsp low carb chocolate chips

For Topping:

- 2 tbsp Keto eggnog
- 2 tsp cinnamon powder

Directions

1. Heat up the waffle maker.
2. Add all the chaffles ingredients to a small mixing bowl and stir until well combined.
3. Add half of the batter into the waffle maker and cook it for approx. 4-5 minutes until golden brown. When the first one is completely cooked, cook the second one.
4. Set aside for 1-2 minutes.

5. Top the chaffle with keto eggnog and sprinkle with cinnamon powder.
6. Serve and enjoy!

Maple Syrup Crispy Chaffle

Preparation: 5 minutes | Cooking: 8 minutes | Servings: 2 chaffles

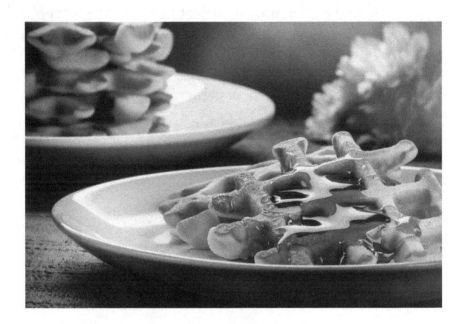

Ingredients

- 1 large egg, beaten
- ¼ cup parmesan cheese, shredded
- ½ cup mozzarella cheese, shredded
- 2 tbsp unsweetened maple syrup for topping

Directions

1. Heat up the waffle maker.

2. Add all the chaffles ingredients except for parmesan cheese to a small mixing bowl and combine well.

3. Now, pour half of the batter into the waffle maker, sprinkle with 1-2 tbsp of shredded parmesan cheese and cook for 4 minutes until golden brown. Repeat now with the rest of the batter to make another chaffle.

4. Let cool for 3 minutes to let chaffles get crispy.

5. Top the chaffles with keto maple syrup.

6. Serve with coconut flour and enjoy!

White Choco Lemon Chaffle

Preparation: 5 minutes | Cooking: 8 minutes | Servings: 2 chaffles

Ingredients

For Chaffles

- 1 large egg, beaten
- ½ tbsp butter, melted
- ½ tbsp softened cream cheese
- 1 tbsp unsweetened white chocolate chips
- 1 tbsp almond flour
- 1 tsp coconut flour
- 1 tbsp sweetener
- ¼ tsp baking powder
- ¼ tsp vanilla extract

For Lemon Icing:

- 2 tbsp sweetener
- 4 tsp heavy cream
- 1 tsp lemon juice
- Fresh lemon zest

Directions

1. Heat up the waffle maker.

2. Add all the chaffles ingredients to a small mixing bowl and stir until well combined.
3. Pour now half of the batter into the waffle maker and cook for 4 minutes. Repeat now with the rest of the batter to prepare the other chaffle.
4. Let cool for 3 minutes to let chaffles get crispy.
5. Combine in a mixing bowl the sweetener, heavy cream, lemon juice and lemon zest. Pour over the chaffles.
6. Serve and enjoy!

Cherry Chocolate Chaffle

Preparation: 4 minutes | Cooking: 8 minutes | Servings: 2 chaffles

Ingredients

- ½ cup shredded mozzarella cheese
- 1 tbsp almond flour
- 1 egg, beaten
- ¼ tsp cinnamon
- ½ tbsp sweetener
- 1 tbsp low carb chocolate chips
- 1 tbsp dark sweet cherries, halved

Directions

1. Heat up the waffle maker.
2. Add now all the ingredients to a small mixing bowl and stir until well combined.
3. Add half of the batter into the waffle maker and cook it for approx. 4-5 min. When the first one is completely done cooking, cook the second one.
4. Set aside for 1-2 minutes.
5. Serve and enjoy!

Cherries Chaffle

Preparation: 5 minutes | Cooking: 8 minutes | Servings: 2 chaffles

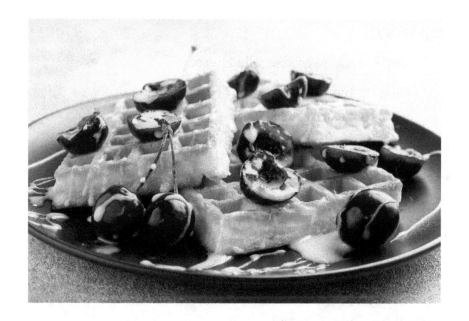

Ingredients

For Chaffles

- 1 large egg, beaten
- ½ cup mozzarella cheese, shredded
- ¼ tsp sweetener

For Topping:

- 2 tbsp dark sweet cherries, halved
- 2 tbsp keto whipped heavy cream

- 2 tsp sweetener

Directions

1. Heat up the waffle maker.
2. Add all the chaffles ingredients to a small mixing bowl and stir until well combined.
3. Pour now half of the batter into the waffle maker and cook for 4 minutes, until brown. Now, repeat with the rest of the batter to make another chaffle.
4. Let cool for 3 minutes to let chaffles get crispy.
5. Spread the chaffles with whipped heavy cream, add cherries and sprinkle with sweetener.
6. Serve and enjoy!

Ricotta Lemon Chaffle

Preparation: 5 minutes | Cooking: 8 minutes | Servings: 2 chaffles

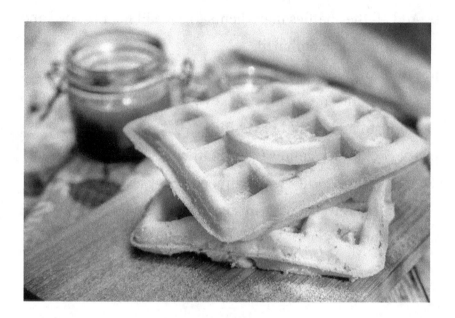

Ingredients

- 1 large egg, beaten
- ½ cup skim ricotta cheese
- 1 tbsp almond flour
- ½ tsp baking powder
- ½ tsp fresh lemon zest
- ½ tsp fresh lemon juice

Directions

1. Heat up the waffle maker.
2. Add now all the ingredients to a small mixing bowl and stir until well combined.
3. Pour now half of the batter into the waffle maker and cook for 4 minutes until golden brown. Now, repeat with the rest of the batter to make another chaffle.
4. Let cool for 3 minutes to let chaffles get crispy.
5. Serve and enjoy!

Pumpkin Cheesecake

Cooking: 15 Minutes | Servings: 2

Ingredients

For chaffle:

- 1 egg
- 1/2 tsp vanilla
- 1/2 tsp baking powder, gluten-free
- 1/4 tsp pumpkin spice
- 1 tsp cream cheese, softened
- 2 tsp heavy cream
- 1 tbsp Swerve
- 1 tbsp almond flour
- 2 tsp pumpkin puree
- 1/2 cup mozzarella cheese, shredded

For filling:

- 1/4 tsp vanilla
- 1 tbsp Swerve
- 2 tbsp cream cheese

Directions

1. Preheat your mini waffle maker.
2. In a small bowl, mix all chaffle Ingredients.

3. Spray waffle maker with cooking spray.
4. Pour half batter in the hot waffle maker and cook for 3-5 minutes. Repeat with the remaining batter.
5. In a tiny bowl, combine all filling Ingredients.
6. Spread Ming mixture between two chaffles and place in the fridge for 10 minutes.
7. Serve and enjoy.

Nutrition: Calories 107, Fat 7.2 g, Carbohydrates 5 g, Sugar 0.7 mg, Sodium 207 mg, Potassium 15mg, Total Carbohydrate 1 g, Dietary Fiber 1 g, Protein 10 g, Total Sugars 1 g,